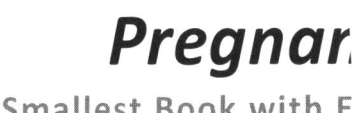

Rewritten and Updated 2nd Edition

Dr. Shahriar Mostafa
MBBS, MPH

ALL RIGHTS RESERVED

Copyright 2016 Dr. Shahriar Mostafa

This ebook is licensed for your personal enjoyment only. This ebook may not be re-sold or given away to other people. Thank you for respecting the hard work of this author.

DEDICATION

<u>I like dedicate this book to my wife Musfica Rahman Nila</u>

Thank you for giving me an angle Wafi Bin Shahriar, My son.

Preface

If you are pregnant or trying to conceive at first I like to congratulate you. Pregnancy is a life changing event. A new life growing inside you is a feeling impossible to describe. The decision to conceive and take up the responsibility of a baby needs a lot of love and courage. As soon as you become pregnant your baby becomes your life. A mother can and would do anything for the baby. Diabetes is a special condition that may happen during pregnancy. The occurrence of this condition is increasing worldwide. Diabetes during pregnancy is becoming a common condition, making it a concern worldwide.

Previously diagnosed diabetic mothers or newly diagnosed gestational diabetic mother has an increased chance of complications during pregnancy and birth. So, we need to plan and prepare for the worst and hope for the best. This book will help you plan and continue your pregnancy safely with diabetes.

If a single pregnancy is helped through this book and its' information, that is the biggest success of this book. The biggest success for me.

Note

This book is not a prescription from doctor. Do not change, increase, start or skip any ongoing treatment without consulting your doctor.

Please visit the following Facebook page and hit like. I will send you every update / edition of this book (eBook only, not printed) completely free.

Facebook Page of Pregnancy & Diabetes

The book will be updated regularly. You can send an email to dr.shahriar@doctor.com "GDM" in subject line. I will email you every update / edition of this book (eBook only, not printed) completely free as thanks for buying this book.

Feel free to Email any question, suggestion or mistake in the book to dr.shahriar@doctor.com "GDM" in subject line. I will answer your questions.

I humbly request you to write a review if you like or dislike this book. It will help me to improve the book. I will mention and add your positive review in future editions of this book.

Click to Review

Thank you for your time.

Acknowledgement

I like to thank Dr. Abdur Rashid MD(Apu) for giving his valuable time to edit this book. Dr. Abdur Rashid is a certified diabetologist. Treating patients successfully for more than 8 years.

Contents

Preface 4
Note 5
Acknowledgement 6
Introduction 10
What is Blood Sugar or Blood Glucose? 12
The journey of carbohydrate within our body. 12
What is diabetes? 13
What is Gestational Diabetes Mellitus or Diabetes of pregnancy? 13
What happens in gestational diabetes? 13
Who gets GDM? 14
How diabetes affects your pregnancy? 15
When to see your doctor? 16
What is the target blood glucose level for a diabetic mother before pregnancy? 16
Recommended visit schedule for a healthy pregnancy? 17
What happens during prenatal visits? 18
Blood and other tests in pregnancy? 20
Diagnosis of GDM? 21
What is kick count? 23
How much weight gain is good in pregnancy? 24
Effect of GDM on the baby? 24
What is the effect of GDM on the mother? 25
Effect of pregnancy on mother with Type 1 or Type 2 diabetes? 26
Effect of diabetes on the baby in Type 2 or Type 1 diabetic mother? 27

How to lower the risk of complications of pregnancy with diabetes (Type 1 or Type 2)? 27

What are the alarming signs of GDM? 28

Treatment options for GDM? 29

Can we lower the chance of getting GDM? 30

Monitoring of blood glucose at home. 30

Steps to check blood glucose at home? 31

Apps for keeping the record of your diabetes? 32

Goals of Gestational Diabetes Treatment. 33

Insulin, what are the types of insulin? 34

What type of insulin do you need for diabetes of pregnancy? 35

How your insulin dose is calculated? 36

How to store insulin? 36

How to give an insulin injection? 37

How to decrease pain when giving insulin? 38

Diabetic ketoacidosis or DKA? 39

How do DKA occur? 39

What is the cause of DKA? 40

How to recognize DKA? 41

Hypoglycemia diagnosis, and treatment? 41

Cause of hypoglycemia? 42

Types of Hypoglycemia and treatment? 42

Glucagon injection for hypoglycemia? 43

Food for gestational diabetes? 44

Tips on food. 45

What is Glycemic Index (GI) of food? 46

Physical Activity with GDM 47

Items you should keep handy during pregnancy with diabetes? 47

After Birth. 48
What to do After History of GDM? 49
Why focus on screening? 50
Future pregnancies 50
Pregnancy with Type 1 or Type 2 diabetes. 50
Breast feeding with diabetes. 51
What supplements should you take? 52
Can you use artificial sweetener during pregnancy? 53
GDM with hypertension...53
Advice on travel with pregnancy and diabetes? 54
Tips for Diabetic mother 54
Conclusion...56
Other Books by Dr. Shahriar Mostafa 57

Introduction

As soon as you learn that you are pregnant your life changes. The love you feel for your child is boundless.

In the course of pregnancy, some of you will be diagnosed with a condition called Gestational Diabetes or the diabetes of pregnancy. As soon as you know from your doctor or healthcare personnel that you have diabetes of pregnancy (Gestational Diabetes) you become terrified. Thousand and thousand questions pop up in your mind.

- What happens in Gestational Diabetes?
- How to control it?
- What's causing it?
- Why did it happen to me?

Your doctor will explain the condition to you but briefly. You will get a lot of leaflets and booklets on Gestational Diabetes(GDM). Also, you will find a thousand websites with million pages. From this ocean of information what you really need to know is difficult to find. And it's time-consuming.

This Book can help.

This book gives you a complete picture on GDM (Gestational Diabetes mellitus). It also gives information on pregnancy with type 1 or type 2 diabetes. If you are a pregnant mother with or without diabetes this book gives all the information you need to protect you and your baby from the complications of GDM or other types of Diabetes.

The main purpose of this book is to save time.

This book is intentionally kept small. You can finish it in 1 hour. In just 1 hour you will have all important information on diabetes of pregnancy (Gestational Diabetes) and pregnancy with previously diagnosed type 1 or type 2 diabetes. It is written in question and answer format; to make the reading easy. From Contents page, you can find the answers to questions you want to know. You will know what to ask your doctor, when you visit, what are the emergency situations when you need immediate treatment.

After skimming through, you should read the whole book. I hope you like this book and information provided here helps you.

Please tell your friends, family and coworkers about it. It's a must read if you are planning for pregnancy.

What is the worldwide condition of gestational diabetes?

The occurrence of GDM is increasing at an alarming rate worldwide. Latest data shows 3 to 5 % pregnant mothers develop GDM during the course of pregnancy.

According to CDC (Center for Diseases Control, USA), GDM occurs 1 in every 20 pregnancies.

What is Blood Sugar or Blood Glucose?

To understand diabetes, you need to know about blood sugar. Main source of sugar or blood glucose in our body is the food we eat. The food we eat contains many substances. After eating, food is broken down into simple forms that our body can use. When food is broken into simple forms we get three major substances. Glucose or Sugar from Carbohydrate (rice, pasta, bread etc.). Fat from oil, butter etc. Protein from meat, milk egg etc.

For diabetes, the carbohydrate or sugar part is important.

The journey of carbohydrate within our body.

Carbohydrate starts its transformation from our mouth to stomach and continue in intestine. Inside our gut food is mashed. Mixed with enzymes and acid and broken down into simple sugar or glucose.

Glucose is the fuel used by our body to do everything we do and keep us alive. From our Gut glucose is absorbed into the blood. Blood carries and delivers this glucose to every cell of our body.

But glucose can't get inside every cell straight from the blood. For glucose to get inside our cells we need insulin. Insulin works as a key for glucose to be transported inside the cells of our body.

What is diabetes?

Insulin is a hormone, made in our body by an organ called the pancreas. To metabolize the food, we eat insulin is essential. If pancreas could not make insulin. Or if your cells do not unlock its doors with insulin, a condition called insulin resistance. Glucose stays in the blood. This increased glucose level in blood is called hyperglycemia. When hyperglycemia is persistent or blood glucose is high all the time we call the condition Diabetes.

What is Gestational Diabetes Mellitus or Diabetes of pregnancy?

When you have persistent high blood glucose during the late phase of pregnancy (after 22 weeks) with no previous history of diabetes the condition is called Gestational Diabetes.

If you have persistent high blood glucose in an early phase of pregnancy (before 22 weeks) then it is not gestational diabetes, most likely it is previously undetected type 2 diabetes.

What happens in gestational diabetes?

You may think GDM occur if you take more sugar, but the cause is very different. There are multiple factors working simultaneously to cause GDM. It occurs due to;

More Hormone During pregnancy, your body makes more hormones. These extra hormones are needed to support the pregnancy and the growing baby. High levels of pregnancy hormones cause your blood glucose level to rise. This rise in blood glucose causes gestational diabetes.

Insulin Resistance Sometimes, insulin does not work effectively. Normally Insulin work as a key to open the doors of your cells for glucose to enter. But sometimes insulin cannot transfer glucose from the blood to cells. The cells of your body block insulin from entering. This condition is medically termed as insulin resistance. Physiological changes in your body during pregnancy cause Insulin resistance.

In Insulin resistance, glucose stays in the blood and causes hyperglycemia (high level of glucose in blood) leading to Diabetes.

Initially Insulin resistance increases your body's need for insulin. If your pancreas can't make enough insulin then glucose can't enter your cells. Glucose stays in blood and you develop gestational diabetes mellitus or diabetes of pregnancy.

All pregnant women show some level of insulin resistance during the late phase of pregnancy (after 22 weeks). But it does not reach too high level to cause diabetes.

Obesity Another reason insulin may not work properly is having excess body fat. The more body fat you have, the less likely it is that your insulin will work properly.

Who gets GDM?

Not everyone of us gets GDM. Extensive studies are done to discover what is causing GDM. Most of the results indicate obesity. So, Obesity is the major risk factor for GDM. Due to lifestyle obesity is affecting more of us, and it's becoming a difficult to control the condition.

Obesity is measured by a scale called BMI or Body Mass Index. BMI uses weight and height to classify obesity. An overweight person with a Body Mass Index or BMI 25 or more are getting GDM more. It's because you will need more insulin during pregnancy if your BMI is 25 or more. If pancreas, the insulin producing organ of the body fails to supply more insulin for the increased demand, GDM occurs.

If you have the previous history of GDM then usually you get GDM in subsequent pregnancies.

There is also a genetic risk of developing GDM. So, if you have siblings with Type 1 or Type 2 Diabetes, the chance of getting GDM is high.

There is a condition where blood glucose level is high, but not high enough to be labeled as diabetes. This condition is called prediabetes. If you were pre-diabetic before pregnancy most likely you will develop GDM during pregnancy.

As genetic factor has a role in getting GDM, African American, American Indian, Asian American, Hispanic/Latino, or Pacific Islander Americans have increased tendency to develop GDM.

Patient of a hormonal disorder called polycystic ovary syndrome has increased chance of developing GDM.

How diabetes affects your pregnancy?

Diabetes before or during pregnancy can cause multiple problems, such as;

- It can increase complications of diabetes, such as diabetes-related heart, eye or kidney diseases.

- Increase chance of birth defects.
- Increase risk of miscarriage (loss of the baby before 22 weeks) or stillborn (baby dies in the womb after 22 weeks)

Don't get nervous with all these negative information, all of these complications occur when your diabetes is not controlled. So, remember for a safe pregnancy your number 1 priority is controlling diabetes.

When to see your doctor?

If you are a diagnosed diabetic patient (type 1 or type 2) you have to see your doctor as soon as you plan to have a baby. It's because diabetes itself may cause difficulty in conception. Some drugs that you might be taking for Type 1 or Type 2 Diabetes needs to be changed as they may not be used during pregnancy or when trying to conceive.

It's always best to visit your doctor when start planning for pregnancy, even if there is no previous history of diabetes, but you have risk factors for diabetes such as obesity, family history present. Doctor will run some tests to see if you are diabetic or prediabetic.

All pregnancies are not planned, unplanned pregnancy occurs commonly. In case of an unplanned pregnancy if you have risk factors of diabetes present, you should visit your doctor as soon as you know that you are pregnant. If you think or feel like you may be pregnant, do a home pregnancy test. If the home pregnancy checking kit shows positive result consult your doctor immediately.

What is the target blood glucose level for a diabetic mother before pregnancy?

If you have diabetes (type 1 or type 2) and planning to have a baby, you must control your blood glucose level first. This is because a baby's brain, heart, kidneys, and lungs develop in the first 8 weeks of pregnancy. High blood glucose levels are especially harmful during this very early stage of conception.

Your target blood glucose level should be;

- Before meals and fasting 80 to 110 mg/dL (4.4 to 6.1 mmol/L) and
- 2 hours after meal 100 to 155 mg/dL (5.6 to 8.6 mmol/L).

Recommended visit schedule for a healthy pregnancy?

Seeing your doctor regularly can help you overcome any complication of GDM.

How many times you have to see your doctor throughout the pregnancy depends on your physical condition and the condition of the baby. It also varies in countries with different healthcare systems. As a general rule, you need to see your doctor at

- <u>Weeks 4 to 28</u>: 1 visit every month (1st 7 months)
- <u>Weeks 28 to 36</u>: 1 prenatal visit every 2 weeks (7 to 9 months)
- <u>Weeks 36 to 40</u>: 1 prenatal visit every week (from 9 months up to delivery)

- Your doctor may increase the number of visits if there is any risk factor of diabetes present.
- <u>Age 35 and more</u>. After age 35, you have an increased chance of having complications. So, you may have to visit your doctor more often.
- <u>Preexisting health problems</u>. If you have a history of diabetes or high blood pressure, or any chronic illness, your doctor will probably want to see you more often.

During prenatal visits, your doctor will look for complications that can occur in pregnancy with diabetes. These complications include

- Preeclampsia
- Pregnancy-related high blood pressure
- Increasing weight of the baby beyond normal weight
- Gestational diabetes.

If you develop any complication, you may need to visit your doctor more often so your doctor can keep close tabs on your health.

Risk of preterm labor. If you have a history of preterm labor or a premature birth, or if you start showing signs of preterm labor, your doctor will want to monitor you more closely.

What happens during prenatal visits?

What happens during prenatal visits varies, depending on how far along you are in your pregnancy and healthcare policy of your country.

Schedule your first prenatal visit as soon as you think you are pregnant, or you have confirmed your pregnancy with a home pregnancy test.

<u>The First Visit</u>

Your first prenatal visit will probably be scheduled sometime after your eighth week of pregnancy. Usually You will feel that you are pregnant around the 8th week after conception. You can visit early if You are planning for pregnancy and missed your regular menstruation. And pregnancy is confirmed it with a home pregnancy test.

If you have had problems with a pregnancy in the past or have symptoms such as spotting or bleeding, stomach pain, or severe nausea and vomiting. Visit your doctor immediately.

Because your first visit will be your longest visit, allow plenty of time.

During the visit, you can expect your health care provider to do the following:

- Answer your questions. This is the best time to ask questions and share any concerns you may have. It's best to Keep a written list of your quarries with you.

During 1st visit your doctor will;

- Check your urine sample for infection and to confirm pregnancy.
- Check your blood pressure, weight, and height.
- Calculate your due date based on your last menstrual cycle and ultrasound exam.
- Ask about your health, including previous conditions, surgeries, or pregnancies.
- Ask about your family health and genetic history.
- You will be asked about your lifestyle, including whether you smoke, drink, or take drugs, and whether you exercise regularly.

Later Prenatal Visits

As your pregnancy progresses, your prenatal visits will vary. During most visits, you can expect your health care provider to do the following:

- Check your blood pressure.
- Measure your weight gain.
- Measure your abdomen to check your developing infant's growth
- Check the fetal heart rate.
- Check your hands and feet for swelling.
- Feel your abdomen to find the fetus's position (later in pregnancy).
- Do tests, such as blood tests or an ultrasound exam.
- Talk to you about your questions or concerns. It's a good idea to write down your questions and bring them with you when visiting your doctor.

Several of these visits will include special tests to check for gestational diabetes (between 24 and 28 weeks) and other conditions, depending on your age and family history. You may be given vaccine needed and recommended by your doctor.

Blood and other tests in pregnancy?

A safe pregnancy needs prevention before any complication occurs. So, you need to go through extensive tests. Your doctor will perform some blood tests:

- To determine your blood type and Rh (Rhesus) factor. Rh factor refers to a protein found in red blood cells. If the mother is Rh-negative (lacks the protein) and the father is Rh-positive (has the protein), the pregnancy requires a special level of care.

- Do a blood count—hemoglobin, hematocrit to see if you have enough hemoglobin to carry oxygen for you and the baby.
- Test for hepatitis B, HIV, rubella, and syphilis.
- Your doctor will do a complete physical exam, including a pelvic exam, gonorrhea and chlamydia cultures, and Pap test to screen for cervical cancer.
- You will need an ultrasound test, depending on the week of pregnancy.
- Genetic testing for screening for Down syndrome, cystic fibrosis and other chromosomal problems.

Please remember This information is based on a general consideration, it may be different according to health care system of your country.

Diagnosis of GDM?

GDM usually shows no symptoms. Most of the time GDM is diagnosed through prenatal screening. Prenatal means before delivery of the baby.

During prenatal visits, Gestational Diabetes Mellitus (GDM) is usually diagnosed by lab investigation. As soon as you become pregnant some tests are done as routine investigation.

- Pregnant women with risk factors will be screened for undiagnosed type 2 diabetes at the first prenatal visit. Your doctor may do a fasting blood glucose & blood glucose 2 hours after breakfast test.
- Pregnant women without any history or risk factor of diabetes is screened at 24-28 weeks for GDM.

For the diagnosis of GDM, any one of the following types of diagnostic tests is done, according to American diabetic association, the strategy to diagnose GDM as follow

"One-Step" Strategy

75g glucose is given orally after fasting overnight or 8 hours. Blood glucose measured of fasting and at 1 hour and 2 hours after taking glucose. This test is done at 24-28 weeks of pregnancy in women not previously diagnosed with any diabetes or GDM.

GDM diagnosis made if blood glucose values are more than:

- Fasting: 92 mg/dL (5.1 mmol/L)
- 1 h: 180 mg/dL (10.0 mmol/L)
- 2 h: 153 mg/dL (8.5 mmol/L)

"Two-Step" Strategy

50-g glucose is given orally. There is no need for fasting before this test. Blood glucose is measured 1 hour after oral glucose. It's done at 24-28 weeks of pregnancy.

If blood glucose at 1 h after oral glucose is ≥140 mg/dL (7.8 mmol/L), proceed to 100-g oral glucose tolerance test, 100g oral glucose test needs fasting overnight or 8 hours.

GDM diagnosis made when two or more blood glucose levels meet or exceed normal levels.

- Fasting: 95 mg/dL or 105 mg/dL (5.3/5.8)
- 1 hour: 180 mg/dL or 190 mg/dL (10.0/10.6)
- 2 hours: 155 mg/dL or 165 mg/dL (8.6/9.2)
- 3 hours: 140 mg/dL or 145 mg/dL (7.8/8.0)

Following is a brief summary on how these tests are done.

Fasting blood glucose test - Done after overnight fasting (No food or drinks for at least 8 hours). You have to give a small amount of blood early in the morning on an empty stomach.

2 hours after 75g glucose OGTT -(Oral Glucose Tolerance Test) In this test after overnight fasting (No food or drinks for at least 8 hours). On an empty stomach, you have to take 75g glucose dissolved in a glass of water. Then after 2 hours, a small amount of blood taken to measure the glucose level in blood.

Other tests are needed and done if you have GDM. Such as,

Ultrasound exams, which use sound waves to make images that show your baby's growth, approximate weight, genetic abnormalities if present and an expected delivery date. Ultrasound exams are completely safe for the baby and can be done multiple time.

A nonstress test, which uses a monitor placed on your abdomen to check whether your baby's heart rate increases as it should when your baby is active.

Kick counts to check the time between your baby's movements.

What is kick count?

One of the most important and easy test you can do for monitoring the well being of your baby is kick count. Kick count checks your baby's movements. It enables the mother to monitor baby's activities and distress.

From 16 and 20 weeks of pregnancy you will begin to feel your baby move. You will be asked to do kick counts every day starting around

26 weeks. By this time, you should be able to clearly feel your baby moving.

Steps to do kick counts;

- Choose the time of day when you feel your baby moves the most. Often this will be after your evening meal.
- Try to check kick counts at the same time every day.
- Lie down on your left side or sit in a comfortable chair.
- Pay attention to your baby's movements.

The first time you feel your baby move, write down the time.

Count every kick or movement until you feel ten movements. Check the time and write it down. Most babies will move ten times or more in one hour.

Take your kick count record sheet every time you visit your doctor.

How much weight gain is good in pregnancy?

The amount of weight gain depends on your weight before pregnancy, your height and physical condition. Your doctor or dietitian will advise you the specific amount of weight you need. As a general rule

- Women who were underweight before pregnancy should gain 28 to 40 pounds
- Women who were normal weight before pregnancy should gain 25 to 35 pounds
- Women who were overweight before pregnancy should gain 15 to 25 pounds
- Women who were obese before pregnancy should limit weight gain upto 11 to 20 pounds

Effect of GDM on the baby?

Having gestational diabetes does not mean your baby will be born with diabetes or birth defects.

When you have GDM you have high blood glucose, during pregnancy your baby gets all the nutrients from your blood. So, it will also have high blood glucose. And as you have diabetes, you can't supply enough insulin needed by the baby.

Baby's pancreas has to make extra insulin to control the high blood glucose it gets from you. As the baby's pancreas makes more insulin to lower the high blood glucose of GDM mother. Just after birth the baby may develop severe Hypoglycemia (low blood glucose) it's a dangerous condition for the baby.

Hypoglycemia may even cause death of the newborn if not treated immediately. The treatment is very simple. We need to supply the newborn glucose immediately after birth. It can be done in any clinic or Hospital.

Another complication of GDM is macrosomia. During fetal period inside the womb, the baby has extra glucose from mother's blood, the extra glucose in baby's blood is converted and stored as fat. So the baby grows larger than normal. It's called macrosomia.

Macrosomia makes normal vaginal delivery difficult and more dangerous for you and your baby. There is increased chance of needing a cesarean section operation to deliver the baby.

After birth, the baby may have breathing problems, a condition called respiratory distress syndrome. This condition occurs more in babies born from mothers suffering from GDM.

The chance of developing neonatal jaundice (yellow discoloration of skin and eyes just after birth) is increased if the mother has GDM.

All these complications sound awful and terrifying, but don't worry. All the complications are preventable and easily treatable. All you need to do is to follow the advice of your doctor and keep your diabetes controlled.

What is the effect of GDM on the mother?

Gestational diabetes may increase your chances of

<u>Preeclampsia</u> – it's a condition where blood pressure is high and loss of protein through urine occur.

<u>Difficult delivery</u> - GDM causes the baby to increase in size, which makes normal delivery impossible so, a surgery called Cesarean section is done to deliver the baby.

<u>Postpartum depression</u> - Mothers with GDM become depressed leading to clinical depression more often than mothers without GDM. Increased stress during pregnancy could be responsible.

<u>Type 2 diabetes</u> - In future, the chance of developing Type 2 diabetes increases with GDM.

Effect of pregnancy on mother with Type 1 or Type 2 diabetes?

During pregnancy, your body goes through multiple changes that creates stress, in known diabetic (Type 1 or Type 2) carries more risk. If untreated, complications of diabetes (type 1 or type 2) may become worse with pregnancy.

If the diabetic mother had preexisting complications of diabetes, such as nephropathy (kidney disease), or retinopathy (eye disease) they may become worse with pregnancy. Monitoring of kidney and eye function must be done throughout pregnancy.

Known diabetic mother gets more episodes of hypoglycemia or low blood glucose during pregnancy. You need to be aware of hypoglycemia. Keep some sugar pills handy all the time. If you feel like low blood glucose with symptoms such as

- Increased sweating
- Dizziness
- Pounding heartbeats

Check your blood sugar immediately.

The chance of preterm labor and premature delivery is increased in known diabetic mothers.

Effect of diabetes on the baby in Type 2 or Type 1 diabetic mother?

If you have uncontrolled diabetes, then it may cause the baby to grow larger than normal. This will complicate the delivery and may require surgery.

There is a risk of death of the baby soon after birth or still born.

How to lower the risk of complications of pregnancy with diabetes (Type 1 or Type 2)?

As you have read early the risk of complications increases during pregnancy if you have type 1 or 2 diabetes. If you are a known diabetic, you need to follow some rules to reduce the risk of developing complications during pregnancy.

<u>Plan your pregnancy</u> – as there are risks involving pregnancy with diabetes, you must plan your pregnancy. Consult your doctor as you start planning for pregnancy.

<u>Control your blood glucose</u> – if your blood glucose level is high most of the time, you should avoid pregnancy until you have a good control. Usually your doctor would do a blood test called HbA1c, which shows overall blood glucose control in last 3 months.

<u>Start Supplements</u> – your doctor will prescribe vitamin supplements and folic acid tablet as soon as you start planning for pregnancy. During early weeks of pregnancy Folic acid is essential to prevent neural tube defect in the baby.

Do not be too worried if you got pregnant without planning. We sure can control diabetes and Prevent complications with effort. Just visit your doctor immediately.

What are the alarming signs of GDM?

Some symptoms and signs in GDM need immediate attention and consultation with a doctor. As these Alarming signs indicate major complication. And you need to be alert for them. The alarming signs of complication are;

- A severe headache - may indicate high blood pressure, preeclampsia or even stroke.
- Your baby moves less or more than normal- indicate distress of the baby, could be due to poor oxygen supply to the baby.
- Severe swelling of face, fingers or feet
- Blurry vision with or without a headache
- Pain or burning when you urinate
- Fever
- Backache or period-like cramps that come and go
- Severe pain in any part of your body that does not go away
- Any spotting of red blood from your vagina (the birth canal)
- Blister or sore in your vaginal area
- Smelly, thick or yellow mucous from your vagina

If you have any of these symptoms anytime throughout the pregnancy, you should contact your doctor as soon as possible for a consultation.

Treatment options for GDM?

Treatment of gestational diabetes focuses mainly on nutrition therapy, exercise, and glucose monitoring aiming for controlling blood glucose. Most of the time GDM is controlled with lifestyle modification only.

To control diabetes (Type 1 & Type 2), we have oral medications and insulin. Oral medicines are taken as pill or capsules Sometimes multiple times a day with or without food. You may have to take multiple groups of oral medicine to control high blood glucose. But these medicines are not usually used in pregnancy. They are not used because there is not enough study to confirm their safety in pregnancy.

Study is difficult to do because who would take risk or permit to study the effect of a drug on her fetus. As there is not enough data on the long-term effect of oral diabetes medicine with pregnancy it's avoided unless absolutely necessary.

Insulin is the preferred treatment for management of diabetes in pregnancy when diet or lifestyle change can't control high blood sugar.

Insulin needs to be used with close monitoring because the requirement of insulin changes rapidly throughout pregnancy. You may need to adjust the dose frequently.

As a general rule in the first trimester, there is often a decrease in total daily dose of insulin. In the second trimester, rapidly increasing insulin resistance needs a weekly or biweekly increase in insulin dose.

Due to the complexity of insulin management in pregnancy, you should visit a specialized center that deals with diabetes with pregnancy or GDM. If this resource is not available, then your doctor can adjust the dose and advise.

Can we lower the chance of getting GDM?

If you are planning for pregnancy, you should take some preventive measure to lower the chance of GDM. All the research shows there is a strong link between obesity and GDM. You can lower this risk,

- First, if you are an obese person then try to lose some weight.
- Start a weight loss workout. Burning calories with exercise is a good way to lose weight.

- Best if you talk with a dietitian and get a plan to reduce weight.

The diet and exercise to lose weight should be discontinued as soon as you become pregnant. For a healthy baby, you need to gain some weight during pregnancy. Your doctor will advise if you need to follow a diet and exercise plan during pregnancy.

Your doctor will tell you how much weight gain and physical activity during pregnancy is safe for you.

Monitoring of blood glucose at home.

Monitoring blood glucose level in the blood is important. You need to check your blood glucose often to see the effect of treatment.

Dose adjustment of insulin also needs blood glucose level, so you need to monitor blood glucose level regularly at home.

Getting pricked with Lancet or syringe is painful. But there is no better working alternative yet. You cannot guess the blood glucose level without a test. Only if the blood glucose level is low you can tell it, but even then, you can't tell how low it is.

Lab test result for blood glucose is almost same using glucometer at home. Glucometer test from the finger blood may vary only 10% of a lab test.

You must maintain a log of your blood glucose level with date, time, condition (empty stomach or after food) and blood glucose level. There are now apps available for iOS, android, and windows to easily maintain a diabetes log.

Steps to check blood glucose at home?

It's very easy to monitor blood sugar using a home testing device. Start the task of home blood glucose monitoring with making the meter ready.

- Insert the strip in the glucose meter.
- If possible, wipe the finger with an alcohol pad or disinfectant.
- Prick finger to get 1 drop of blood.
- Give the blood on the strip. In a few seconds, the meter will display current blood glucose level.

Do finger prick on the side of the finger where pain sensation is low. If available, use low pain lancet. It will reduce pain. Use alternate finger every time. If blood does not come after finger prick by the Lancet, a gentle squeeze of the finger will help.

Carefully store glucometer strips. Only 2-hour exposure to air will damage the strip. Blood glucose level from finger prick is better than blood from other sites (heel, ear lobe etc.)

Apps for keeping the record of your diabetes?

Monitoring and keeping the record of your blood glucose level is easy now. There are many apps for iPhone, iPad, Android and Windows. To give you an initial idea of these apps, I have reviewed two of the apps. You can use these apps or find one of your choices.

Diabetes: M

Designed for smartphones and tablets this application is intended to help diabetics to manage better their diabetes and keep it under control. Users can log their values in this diary and keep the records with them all the time. The application tracks almost all aspects of the diabetes treatment and provides detailed reports, charts, and statistics to share via the email with the supervising physician. It provides various tools to the diabetics, so they can find the trends in blood glucose levels and allows users to calculate normal and prolonged insulin boluses using its highly effective, top-notch bolus calculator.

"Diabetes: M" can analyze the values from the imported data from various glucometers and insulin pumps via the exported files from their respective diabetes management software systems.

Supports Android Wear smartwatches. The app is available in Android play store and iTunes store.

mySugr Diabetes Logbook

mySugr Logbook app is a charming diabetes tracker for blood glucose, bolus, basal, food, carbs, meds, pills, weight, a1c and more. It makes your diary useful in everyday life with playful elements and immediate feedback through your diabetes monster! Get motivated and involved in your diabetes therapy, today!

— No. 1 diabetes logbook app in 6 countries

— Most popular diabetes logbook app in the world based on five-star reviews and ratings

— Winner of Germany's "Focus Diabetes" 'Best Apps for People with Diabetes' award

Our motto: We make diabetes suck less!

FEATURES/ADD-ONS:

• Designed for type 1 & type 2 diabetes

• Quick and easy logging (meals, meds, BG's, and more)

• Personalized logging screen (add, remove, and reorder fields)

- Estimated HbA1c - so there are no more nasty surprises

- CGM data integration via CSV import (only available in German and English speaking countries)

- Daily, weekly, monthly analysis (and more)

- Exciting challenges for personal therapy goals

Goals of Gestational Diabetes Treatment.

When you want to control your blood glucose for a healthy and safe pregnancy, you have to set certain goals for your blood glucose level. These goals will show your effort and help you measure your achievement. According to these goals, you can modify your lifestyle and treatment plan.

Gestational Diabetes Mellitus have the following blood glucose targets:

- Before food or Fasting blood glucose target is 95mg/dL (5.3mmol/L)
- One-hour after food target blood glucose level 140 mg/dL (7.8 mmol/L)
- Two-hour after food the target blood glucose level 120 mg/dL (6.7 mmol/L)

For women with preexisting type 1 diabetes or type 2 diabetes who became pregnant, the following are recommended blood glucose target.:

- Premeal, bedtime, and overnight target glucose level 60–99 mg/dL (3.3–5.4 mmol/L)
- Peak after meal glucose level 100–129 mg/dL (5.4–7.1 mmol/L)
- HbA1C ,6.0%

These targets and goals are not set in stone. The blood sugar goal depends on your physical condition and other factors. Your doctor will help you decide which target blood glucose level is best for you.

Insulin, what are the types of insulin?

Since its discovery in 1921. Insulin has become the most prescribed drug in history.

As a drug, Insulin is made from animals (cow, pig etc.) or from bacteria genetically engineered to make insulin same as human insulin. Some manufactured insulin is modified to work better. Those modified insulins are called insulin analog.

Insulin is given by injection. If insulin taken by mouth, it gets broken down, digested and becomes inactive in our stomach. That's why insulin you need to get it through an injection.

Insulin Injection is given just under the skin. If we give insulin injection in the vein or muscle it works for a very short time. That's why it is given under skin so it's absorbed slowly and work for a long time.

There are many types of insulin. Following are the types we usually use regularly

- Rapid Acting Insulin as the name implies, this type of insulin works within 15 min of injection and works up to 4 hours.
- Short-acting insulin or regular insulin starts working in 30 minutes. It continues work up to 6 hours.
- Intermediate-acting Insulin - gets into blood in 2 hours. And works up to 18 hours.
- Long-acting insulin reaches blood in 3 or 4 hours after injection. And works up to 24 hours.

- Also, there is mixed insulin containing rapid acting insulin analog and medium or long acting insulin. Given before meals. They start to work 30 minutes after injection and works a long time.

What type of insulin do you need for diabetes of pregnancy?

The type and dose of insulin must be advised by the doctor. It can be harmful if you get an insulin injection in veins or muscle or in large doses. Never change your treatment plan without consulting your doctor or health care professional.

In general, most of the GDM mothers need multiple doses of insulin injection. To reduce the chance of hypoglycemia, insulin analogs are used.

How your insulin dose is calculated?

The amount of insulin needed is different for different persons. So, you need to consult your doctor to adjust your insulin dose.

The aim of insulin treatment is to mimic normal insulin production without diabetes.

This is done using:

- Basal insulin - This deals with the glucose produced by your liver. If you skip a meal, your basal insulin alone should be able to keep your blood glucose levels stable.

- Bolus insulin- While basal insulin influences your blood glucose levels in between meals, it's the bolus (fast-acting) insulin that deals with the carbohydrate contained in any food and drink you have.

But remember you should never change (increase or decrease) your insulin dose without consulting your doctor or health care provider. Your doctor will calculate how much insulin needed (Dose). Also, the doctor will tell you how many times insulins is needed and which type of insulin needed.

How to store insulin?

Keep the insulin you are currently using at room temperature. It's best to keep it under 25 degrees. Injection of cold insulin is painful.

- If you keep your regular use insulin in a freezer. Be sure to take out insulin from freezer more than 30 minutes before getting injected. Keep it at room temperature for at least 30 minutes.
- Store insulin for a long period at 4 to 6-degree temperature.
- Do not completely freeze insulin.
- Never heat insulin or keep it beside the source of heat (oven, TV, locked car, radiator etc.)
- For travel, use a special cold bag or use a flask to keep it cold.
- Check the expiration date and color of insulin. If there are clamps or the color changed through the insulin away.

How to give an insulin injection?

Your doctor or diabetes educator will show the proper syringe and show you how to get an insulin injection

Follow these easy steps to give an insulin injection

- Wash your hand.
- Check the insulin bottle for expiring date.
- Check the insulin bottle for clamps, color change. If there is clamps or color change do not give insulin from that vial.
- Wipe the cap of the insulin bottle with an alcohol pad.
- Clean the skin where you will get the injection. With alcohol pad or soap and water.
- Pinch skin and fat with thumb.
- Push the needle into your skin: With your other hand, hold the syringe at a 45-degree angle. Make sure the needle is all the way into the skin.
- Let go of the pinched tissue before you inject the insulin
- Inject the insulin: Press the plunger with your thumb. Use slow and steady push until the insulin is gone.
- Pull out the needle: Pull out the needle at the same angle you put it in. Press your injection site with cotton for a few seconds.
- Throw away your used insulin syringe.

It's best if you use each Insulin syringe only once. The needle of the syringe becomes blunt after repeated use and become painful for you. Throw away used needles and syringes in a hard container. So, that the needles cannot stick through. Close the container with a screw-on cap. Keep the container out of reach of children and pets.

Don't use insulin if:

- Clear insulin has turned cloudy or changed color
- The expiry date has been reached
- Insulin has been frozen or exposed to high temperatures
- Lumps or flakes can be seen

- The vial has been opened for more than 28 days

How to decrease pain when giving insulin?

- Inject insulin at room temperature. If the insulin stored in the refrigerator, remove it 30 minutes before you inject it. Cold insulin injection is painful.
- Remove all air bubbles from the syringe before the injection.
- If you clean your skin with an alcohol pad, wait until it has dried before you inject insulin.
- Relax the muscles at the injection site.
- Avoid changing the direction of the needle during insertion or removal.
- Do not reuse disposable needles. Because needles get blunt and cause pain.
- Try numbing the area of injection by use of an ice cube. Keep the ice cube pressed to skin for 2 minutes just before injection. This works and can reduce the pain significantly.
- Always use a different site to give the injection.

Diabetic ketoacidosis or DKA?

DKA (Diabetic Ketoacidosis) is a dangerous complication of diabetes, the patient may die if DKA is not treated immediately.

DKA usually occurs in patients with Type 1 diabetes, but It can also occur in GDM.

During pregnancy, diabetic ketoacidosis usually occurs in the second and third trimesters because in second and third trimester there is increased insulin resistance.

In pregnancy DKA tends to occur at lower blood glucose levels and more rapidly than in non-pregnant patients often causing a delay in the diagnosis and treatment.

How do DKA occur?

With Gestational diabetes, insulin resistance increases, to overcome this resistance you need more insulin. Your pancreas starts to make more and more insulin for the increased demand.

Eventually the pancreas can't produce adequate amount of insulin as the body needs. Moreover, insulin does not function properly in case of GDM.

All these causes high blood glucose but the cells of our body don't get glucose.

Glucose is the main source of energy for our body to function. Our body needs glucose. In DKA, to meet the energy demand our body starts to breakdown stored Fat of the body. Breakdown of fat provides essential energy, but leads to ketone production. Ketone is a byproduct of fat metabolism and it is harmful for us. With ketone blood becomes acidic, leading to diabetic ketoacidosis.

DKA is a medical emergency and must be treated at a hospital.

What is the cause of DKA?

The cause of DKA in Gestational Diabetes (GDM) includes

- Severe vomiting
- Infection (Pneumonia or lung infection or Urine infection).
- Missed insulin injection
- Trauma
- Stroke
- Some medicines such as corticosteroid therapy and poor management of diabetes.

DKA is a medical emergency, treatment can only be given at hospital / clinic. To confirm DKA a home urine test can be done, which will show deep purple color indicating high level of ketone in the body.

To prevent DKA, you should never miss insulin injection. Monitor signs of DKA.

How to recognize DKA?

DKA or diabetic keto acidosis is a serious condition that needs urgent treatment in hospital setting. It's very important to recognize the symptoms of DKA. Following are some signs of DKA

- Fruity Smell of acetone is a major symptom of diabetic ketoacidosis.
- Sweating
- Cold, clammy skin
- Increased thirst
- Abdominal pain
- Nausea & vomiting
- Confusion or coma.

These are the symptoms of DKA. If you recognize 2 or more of these symptoms check your blood glucose level using glucometer, if possible, check your urine for ketone with a home testing kit. If your blood glucose level is high and there is high ketone in your urine consultant with your doctor immediately.

You should teach your family members or friends who are living with you to recognize symptoms of DKA.

If all this information is stressing you, don't be stressed, DKA is a treatable condition. With immediate treatment, the possibility of harm to you or your baby is very low.

Another complication of all types of diabetes including GDM is Hypoglycemia (low blood glucose).

Hypoglycemia diagnosis, and treatment?

Hypoglycemia or low blood glucose is a short-term complication of diabetes. It is a common but dangerous condition. The good thing is hypoglycemia shows certain symptoms. Which makes it easy to recognize.

Hypoglycemia symptoms start to show as soon as blood glucose level becomes 75 mg/dl or lower. Symptoms include

- Anxiety,
- Irritability
- Numbness in the lips, fingers, and toes.
- Sweating
- Shaking
- Feeling weak or tired
- Racing heart or palpitation

Cause of hypoglycemia?

Most of the time accidentally taking insulin in high dose causes Hypoglycemia. Another cause of hypoglycemia is

- Taking the wrong type of insulin.
- Missed meal or taking a small amount of food
- Too much physical exercise.

Some drugs may lower blood glucose leading to hypoglycemia. Such drugs are Beta blocker for hypertension, Aspirin for a headache.

Mild hypoglycemia is treated with a small portion of food. Take carbohydrate or sugar containing drinks.

Types of Hypoglycemia and treatment?

<u>Moderate Hypoglycemia</u> - When the blood glucose level becomes 65mg/dl or low it's called moderate hypoglycemia. Symptoms include Rapid heartbeat. The sensation of hunger. Sweating and Whiteness or pallor of the skin.

Moderate hypoglycemia needs 4 to 5 glucose tablets or oral glucose. Recheck blood glucose after 20 minutes. If the blood glucose level is still low give more glucose tablet or powder and recheck again.

<u>Sever Hypoglycaemia</u> - When the blood glucose level is less than 55 mg/dl it's called severe hypoglycemia. Symptoms include Confusion and trouble concentrating, Convulsions, Dizziness, Fatigue, Feeling of warmth, and headache, Reduced consciousness or coma, and Slurred speech.

Severe hypoglycemia is a medical emergency. Use a glucagon injection if available and prescribed by your doctor.

There are some common things to do in any type of hypoglycemia or low blood glucose. If the patient is conscious and can take food by mouth. She should be given 3 to 4 glucose tablets or give 15ml or three teaspoons of honey. Recheck blood glucose in 20 minutes. If the blood glucose level is still low, give more glucose tablet or honey.

If the patient is unconscious or unable to take food. Consult your doctor or health care provider.

Instead of glucose tablet (if unavailable). Give sugar containing drinks such as Apple juice or orange juice.

Glucagon injection for hypoglycemia?

Glucagon is a hormone, and it's given in severe hypoglycemia to protect the body.

Glucagon comes in a package contains powder glucagon and water for injection in 2 vials. A syringe with needle is also available.

- First, Check the expiration date of glucagon injection
- Take water from a vial with syringe.
- Inject the water in the powder containing bottle.
- Shake to mix powder glucagon with water.
- Take mixed drug using the syringe and inject into muscle. In hip or upper arm.

You and family members should learn to know the symptoms of hypoglycemia. And how to give the glucagon injection.

You need to have glucagon injection, glucose monitoring device and sugar tablet with you at all time.

Food for gestational diabetes?

Food is a major component in the treatment of GDM. It is important to discuss with a dietitian for a personalized diet plan.

Bread, rice, potatoes, pasta & other starchy foods these are the source of carbohydrate. They give us all the energy we need. But carbohydrate is also the main source of glucose in the blood. You should watch how much carbohydrate you take. 40 to 60 percent of calories of our diet should come from carbohydrate.

Meat, fish, eggs, beans are sources of protein. Proteins are needed to repair and growth of our body. It does not have a direct effect on blood glucose. Protein is the main component of hormones, enzymes and antibodies. 10 to 20 percent of calories of your diet should come from protein. As part of a mixed meal, protein slows the absorption of carbohydrate, which is good for you.

Milk & dairy foods have essential vitamins and minerals. These products have an effect on blood glucose.

Fruit & vegetables contain essential vitamins. For a healthy diet fruit and vegetables are essential.

Tips on food.

Food is part of treatment. It's best to consult with a dietitian to get your personalized diet plan. There are some common tips to help you with your diet.

- Always use low-fat milk, cheese, yogurt and dairy products.
- Use pulses such as peas, beans or lentils to replace or reduce meat.
- Cut and remove visible fat from meat, from poultry product remove skin.
- When cooking, try to drain excess fat from meat before adding spices.
- Try to grill or baking instead frying. Learn low-fat cooking methods.
- Eat carbohydrate that slow to absorb with low glycemic Index.
- Eat pasta, basmati or easy cook rice, grainy bread such as granary, pumpernickel, rye, new potatoes, sweet potato, yam porridge, oats and natural muesli. These foods have a low glycemic index so blood glucose will be low.

- For fat Choose unsaturated fats or oils, such as olive, rapeseed and sunflower oil. These fats will help you to lose weight. You will reach your target cholesterol level with low fat.
- Use less butter, margarine and cheese.
- Eat fish at least once every week.
- Eat one portion of fruit such as 1 apple or banana or any other fruit you like every day.
- Avoid sugary drinks or smoothies.
- Do not take more than 6g of salt per day. Less salt reduces blood pressure and heart disease.

What is Glycemic Index (GI) of food?

You will always be advised to monitor GI of your food. The Glycemic Index (GI) is a way to measure how a particular food affects blood glucose level. It's used for carbohydrate based food only. Slowly absorbed foods have a low GI rating while foods that are more quickly absorbed have a higher rating. Low GI food is good for maintaining your diabetes.

Choosing slowly absorbed carbohydrates with a low GI index, instead of quickly absorbed carbohydrates with higher GI, can help even out blood glucose levels when you have diabetes.

There is a negative side to GI (Glycemic index), it measures one food especially carbohydrate at a time. whereas we eat carbohydrates as part of a meal. Things, such as cooking methods, ripeness of fruits and vegetables and the fat or protein content of a meal will affect the glycemic index of a food.

It's important that if you restrict yourself to eating only low GI foods, your diet will be unbalanced and may be high in fat and calories, leading to weight gain and increasing your risk of heart disease. Do not focus exclusively on GI. Eat a balanced diet with low fat, salt and sugar and containing plenty of fruit and vegetables.

Physical Activity with GDM

Exercise will help you use your excessive blood sugar. Before exercising, talk to your doctor and health care team. They will tell you what exercise is safe for you.

One of the best exercises for pregnant women is walking. Try to walk at least once a day. Do more if you can. Your goal is to walk twenty minutes after each meal. Walking after a meal helps lower your blood glucose.

If your BMI was more than 27 before you became pregnant, you may be advised to take moderate exercise for at least 150 minutes (2 hours and 30 minutes) a week. But remember never start any physical activity or exercise without consulting your doctor.

Items you should keep handy during pregnancy with diabetes?

- Emergency contact information.
- Monitoring equipment (e.g. lancets, meter strips, alcohol, ketone strips, sensor supplies)
- Glucose tablets or other fast-acting forms of
- Carbohydrate to treat hypoglycemia.
- Insulin and related supplies (e.g. insulin syringes and/or pen).
- Ketone monitoring supplies.
- Glucagon kit.

After Birth.

After your baby is delivered, your body begins to recover from the hard work of pregnancy and delivery. New mothers have better blood glucose control in the first few weeks after delivery. But sometimes it's a period of odd blood glucose swings.

Not being able to predict how your body will act may leave you puzzled and upset. It is best to check your blood glucose levels very frequently following delivery to avoid either high or low blood glucose levels until you get an idea of how much insulin your body needs.

You should be aware of the symptoms of high blood glucose (hyperglycemia), which could be a sign your diabetes has returned. These symptoms are:

- Increased thirst
- The need to urinate frequently
- Tiredness

Depending on your glucose levels at diagnosis, you will either have to repeat oral glucose tolerance test (OGTT) or your doctor will arrange a HbA1c test (a marker of your average blood glucose over the preceding 3 months) at 12 weeks after delivery.

If you have type 2 diabetes, your doctor will decide which medication you should start after delivery. You will usually be able to go back to the same medications you were taking before pregnancy, as long as they were controlling your diabetes well. Your diabetes medications need to be modified if you are breastfeeding.

If you have gestational diabetes, there is a very good chance that your diabetes will go away immediately after the delivery. This is especially true if your diabetes was controlled with only a meal plan and exercise during pregnancy. You should continue to check your blood glucose levels for at least several days to make sure your diabetes is actually gone.

Your weight and waist measurement may be monitored and you should be given advice about diet and exercise.

An HbA1c will then be measured at least once a year to check whether or not you have developed type 2 diabetes.

Women with a history of gestational diabetes frequently develop type 2 diabetes later, though, so check with your healthcare team about being checked for type 2 every 1–3 years.

What to do After History of GDM?

After a safe pregnancy and a healthy baby with GDM, you may think that it's time to forget about GDM. But it's not a good idea. You will need regular checkup for diabetes because there is increased risk of having type 2 diabetes after having GDM.

You should be checked for diabetes with 75g glucose OGTT test 6 weeks after delivery, then again 6 months after delivery then again, every 3 years. You should be checked if you start palming for another baby or as soon as you are pregnant.

Why focus on screening?

GDM significantly increases the risk of developing type 2 diabetes later in life. As many as 30 percent of women with a history of GDM will develop diabetes within 15 years.

After a history of GDM screening allows for targeted lifestyle intervention to reduce the risk of developing type 2 diabetes. With type 2 diabetes, screening helps to reduce the risk of complications of diabetes.

So, regular and timely screening for type 2 diabetes is essential for women who have had gestational diabetes. Talk to your health-care provider and be sure you receive regular testing for type 2 diabetes.

Future pregnancies

After having gestational diabetes, you are at increased risk of having gestational diabetes in any future pregnancies.

It's very important to speak to your doctor before planning another pregnancy in the future. In future pregnancies, you have to monitor your blood glucose from the early stage.

Pregnancy with Type 1 or Type 2 diabetes.

Type 1 diabetes

Type 1 diabetes usually starts from childhood. In type one diabetes body does not produce any insulin. So, insulin is given from outside via Injections

If you have type 1 diabetes, pregnancy will affect your insulin treatment plan. During the months of pregnancy, your body's need for insulin will go up. This is especially true during the last three months of pregnancy. The need for more insulin is caused by hormones the placenta makes. The placenta makes hormones that help the baby grow. At the same time, these hormones block the action of the mother's insulin. As a result, your insulin needs will increase.

Type 2 diabetes

In Type 2 diabetes body produces inadequate amounts of insulin.

If you have type 2 diabetes, you too need to plan ahead. If you are taking diabetes pills to control your blood glucose, you may not be able to take them when you are pregnant. Because the safety of using diabetes pills during pregnancy has not been established, your doctor will probably have you switch to insulin right away. Also, the insulin resistance that occurs during pregnancy often decreases the effectiveness of oral diabetes medication at keeping your blood glucose levels in their target range.

Breast feeding with diabetes.

It does not matter what type of diabetes you have (type 1, type 2 or gestational) breastfeeding is safe for your baby. Moreover, it is very helpful for the baby to boost its immunity, gain weight and create a special bond with the mother.

You should breastfeed the baby just after birth. You may continue Breastfeeding up to a year or more. It's best to breastfeed your baby at least for first 3 months, during these months only breast milk is enough for the baby, no additional supplements or food is needed.

After 6 months, your baby will need other foods with breast milk.

If you have type 1 or type 2 diabetes and use either insulin or oral blood glucose lowering medications, it's important to understand the safety of these medications while breastfeeding. Most medications used to treat diabetes can be safely used during breastfeeding. But check with your doctor to find out if your medications can be continued while breastfeeding.

Breastfeeding also helps you lose the weight you gained during pregnancy. But do not try to lose it too quickly.

While you are breastfeeding, it is important that you get the right amounts of fluids, protein, vitamins, and minerals.

Working with your dietitian, you should be able to develop a meal plan that will allow you to achieve gradual weight loss and still be successful at breastfeeding.

Breastfeeding may make your blood glucose level unpredictable. Most of the time you may experience low blood glucose levels due to breastfeeding, try these tips if you feel your blood glucose level is getting low:

Plan to have a snack before or during nursing

Drink enough fluids (plan to sip a glass of water or a caffeine-free drink while nursing)

Keep something to treat low blood glucose nearby when you nurse, so you don't have to stop a feeding to treat low blood glucose levels

What supplements should you take?

During pregnancy, you need extra iron, calcium etc. Essential minerals and vitamins are needed for proper growth of your baby.

You should take iron to help make extra blood for pregnancy and for maintaining the baby's supply of iron.

You must take Folic Acid to prevent birth defects in the brain and spinal cord of the baby.

Take Calcium to build strong bones.

If you are a known diabetic (type 1 or type 2) you should start your vitamin and mineral supplements before pregnancy. As soon as you start planning for pregnancy start a folic acid supplement at least 1 month before you get pregnant.

Vitamin D supplements, studies suggest that having enough vitamin D in your blood may help maintain healthy blood glucose levels. Ask your doctor whether you should take a vitamin D supplement.

Can you use artificial sweetener during pregnancy?

During pregnancy, artificial sweeteners can be used in moderate amounts. If you choose to use sweeteners, talk with your dietitian about how much artificial sweetener you can take.

GDM with hypertension.

GDM is more complicated if you have hypertension (high blood pressure). Target blood pressure during pregnancy is

- Systolic Blood Pressure 110 to 129 mmHg
- Diastolic Blood Pressure 65 to 79 mmHg

Some medicines such as ACE inhibitor ARB used to control your hypertension cannot be used during pregnancy as they can damage the baby.

Safe drugs such as Mthyldopa, Labitelol, Diltiazem, Clonidine etc. are safe to be used in hypertension during pregnancy.

Your doctor will decide which one is best for you.

Advice on travel with pregnancy and diabetes?

Your Gynecologist or doctor will determine if travel is safe for you. There are some tips on stuff you need to carry;

If you take insulin, then take a special insulated bag to carry insulin. Remember not to freeze or make it too hot. Carry glucometer, glucometer strips and lancet, to monitor blood glucose if any emergency occurs. Keep some dry snacks and glucose tablets handy for the treatment of hypoglycemia (low blood glucose) if occur.

Tips for Diabetic mother

- If you are a diabetic woman preparing for pregnancy or a newly diagnosed GDM patient, these tips will help you.
- If you have diabetes before pregnancy, the best time to control your blood glucose is before you get pregnant.
- Keeping your blood glucose as close to normal as possible before and during your pregnancy is the most important thing you can do to stay healthy and have a healthy baby.
- Regular visits with your doctor or health care team, expert in diabetes and pregnancy will help you learn how to use a healthy eating plan, physical activity, and medicine. It will help you to reach your blood glucose targets before and during pregnancy.
- During pregnancy, the safest diabetes medicine is insulin. Some medicines are not safe during pregnancy and should be stopped before you get pregnant. Your doctor can tell you which medicines to stop taking.
- Avoid alcohol or alcohol containing beverages.
- Stop smoking, smoking hampers the oxygen supply of the baby, affecting baby's growth & development.
- Eat healthy diet as advised by your doctor or nutritionist.
- Stay active, choose an activity you are comfortable and approved by your doctor.
- Eat small healthy snacks in between meals.
- If you have repeated vomiting, check your urine for ketones at home (if possible) consult your doctor immediately if urine ketone is positive.

- Learn to give Insulin, Glucagon injection and teach your family member or friends to give injections in case of emergency.
- You can give your baby a healthy start by breastfeeding.

Conclusion

Thank you for reading this book. I wish you a safe pregnancy with a healthy baby. Please write a small review of this book if you can. Share the link of this book on amazon with your friends, family or coworkers, if you think this book can help with their pregnancy.

<u>The End</u>

About the author

I am Dr. Shahriar Mostafa, completed my medical education (MBBS) in 2009. Then completed Master's degree in Public Health in 2013. I have been working in a Medical College Hospital for last 7 years. I want to write simple and small patient education books to reach a larger audience.

Other Books by Dr. Shahriar Mostafa

Diagnosed with Diabetes. Now What!

Smallest Book with Everything You Need to Know

https://www.amazon.com/dp/B01HC0CF26

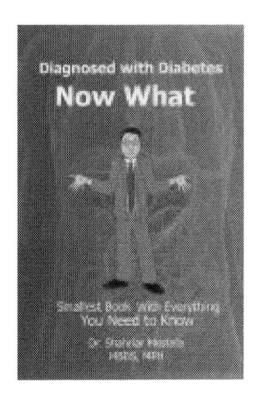

You were living your life to the fullest. Working hard and playing harder. Ignoring symptoms like fatigue, weight loss and increased frequency of urination. Then BAM! Out of the blue you started feeling very sick. You consult with your doctor, he runs some tests and you are diagnosed with diabetes!
Now What!

Should you leave all the things you love to do? Stop eating desserts. Adopt a life of Saints! Should you get panicked and think that's it, this is the end of the road! Well, it's not like that.

This book will help you to keep your diabetes well controlled. It's a small book but packed with information on diabetes you must know. Grab your copy and let's start for a healthy, happy and fulfilling life with Diabetes.

Type One Diabetes:

Smallest book with everything you need to know

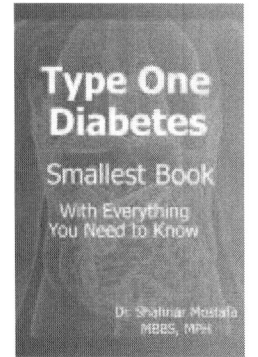

https://www.amazon.com/dp/B01AQOJ21C

As soon as you learn that you or your child has type one diabetes you become terrified. What happens in type one diabetes? What to do to cure it? How to control it? How to explain this to a child? What's causing it? Why did it happen to me? Thousand and thousand questions pop up in your mind. You search the internet which shows a million pages. You ask your health care personal but not satisfied with the answers. You become confused, afraid and angry.

But you don't have to be confused or afraid. You are not alone. Type one diabetes is a common disease. About 350 million people worldwide have diabetes. It is easy to control. It does not keep you from anything the life has to offer. But there is a catch, you have to control type one diabetes all your life.

Type 2 Diabetes: Smallest book with everything you need to know

https://www.amazon.com/dp/B01FUGZASK

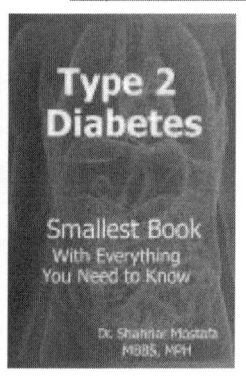

Diabetes is a common disease. About 350 million people worldwide have diabetes. It is easy to control. It does not keep you from anything the life has to offer. But there is a catch, you have to control Diabetes all your life.

This book is small and you do not have to read this book from page one to the end. You can start anywhere and slowly finish it. Use the table of contents to find the topic of your interest and start from there. You can finish this book in just 1 hour. In 1 hour, you will have all important information on Type 2 Diabetes. This book will give the confidence, hope and information to live a normal, happy life with Type 2 Diabetes.

High Blood Pressure: Control With and Without Medicine

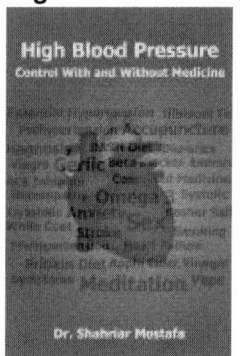

https://www.amazon.com/dp/B01MQHV94K

High blood pressure or Hypertension leading to life-threatening complication is a reality. All the study and data indicate that most of us will get high blood pressure.

For hypertension prevention, you need to be prepared and start preventive measures as early as possible. In this book, I have tried to give all these answers. I have given pro and cons of drug and non-drug (Herbal, Homeopathic, Meditation) treatments proven to be useful for hypertension. Also included and explained treatments that are useless for hypertension.

With information, I hope you can make an informed decision on your treatment plan. And you can also work on prevention of high blood pressure.

Printed in Great Britain
by Amazon